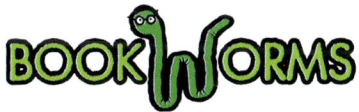

Community Workers

A Dentist's Job

Erika de Nijs

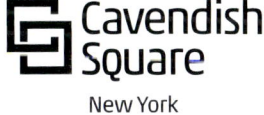

Cavendish Square

New York

Published in 2016 by Cavendish Square Publishing, LLC
243 5th Avenue, Suite 136, New York, NY 10016

Copyright © 2016 by Cavendish Square Publishing, LLC

First Edition

No part of this publication may be reproduced, stored in a retrieval system, or transmitted in any form or by any means—electronic, mechanical, photocopying, recording, or otherwise—without the prior permission of the copyright owner. Request for permission should be addressed to Permissions, Cavendish Square Publishing, 243 5th Avenue, Suite 136, New York, NY 10016. Tel (877) 980-4450; fax (877) 980-4454.

Website: cavendishsq.com

This publication represents the opinions and views of the author based on his or her personal experience, knowledge, and research. The information in this book serves as a general guide only. The author and publisher have used their best efforts in preparing this book and disclaim liability rising directly or indirectly from the use and application of this book.

CPSIA Compliance Information: Batch #WS15CSQ

All websites were available and accurate when this book was sent to press.

Library of Congress Cataloging-in-Publication Data

de Nijs, Erika.
A dentist's job / Erika de Nijs.
pages cm. — (Community workers)
Includes bibliographical references and index.
ISBN 978-1-50260-425-5 (hardcover) ISBN 978-1-50260-424-8 (paperback)
ISBN 978-1-50260-426-2 (ebook)
1. Dentists—Juvenile literature. 2. Teeth—Care and hygiene—Juvenile literature.
3. Dentistry—Vocational guidance—Juvenile literature. I. Title.

RK63.D38 2015
617.6'0232—dc23

2014050271

Editorial Director: David McNamara
Editor: Fletcher Doyle
Copy Editor: Cynthia Roby
Art Director: Jeffrey Talbot
Designer: Alan Sliwinski
Senior Production Manager: Jennifer Ryder-Talbot
Production Editor: Renni Johnson

The photographs in this book are used by permission and through the courtesy of: Vagengeim/shutterstock.com, cover; Maksym Poriechkin/shutterstock.com, 5; Mike Kemp/Getty Images, 7; Pressmaster/shutterstock.com, 9; Rich Legg/Getty Images, 11; Ocskay Bence/shutterstock.com, 13; Ocskay Bence/shutterstock.com, 15; Image Source/Getty Images, 17; Peter Dazeley/Getty Images, 19; KPG_Payless/shutterstock.com, 21.

Printed in the United States of America

Contents

Who Are Dentists? **4**

New Words **22**

Index **23**

About the Author **24**

I am a dentist.

I keep your teeth **healthy**.

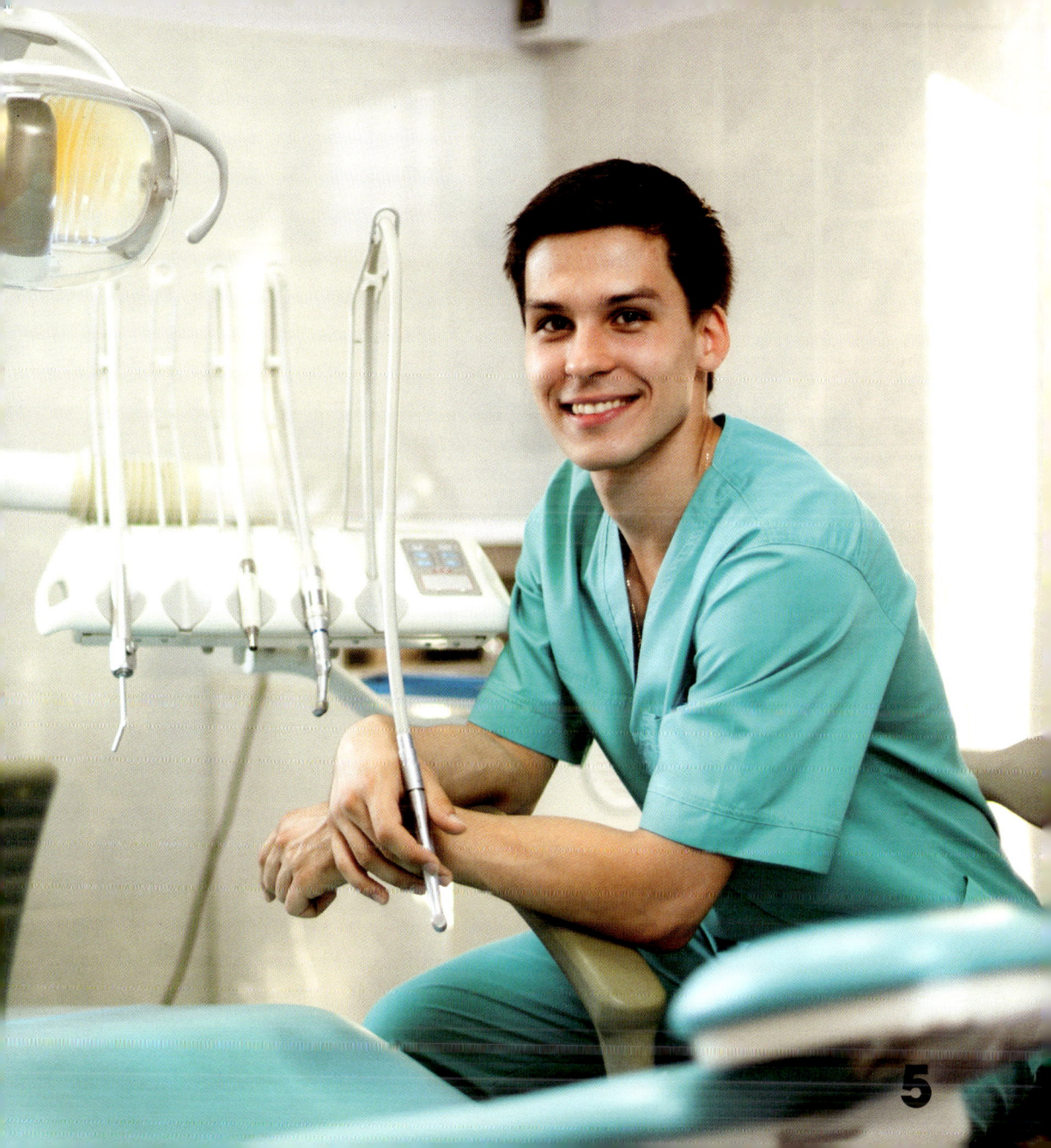

Lean back in the dentist chair.

This helps me clean your teeth.

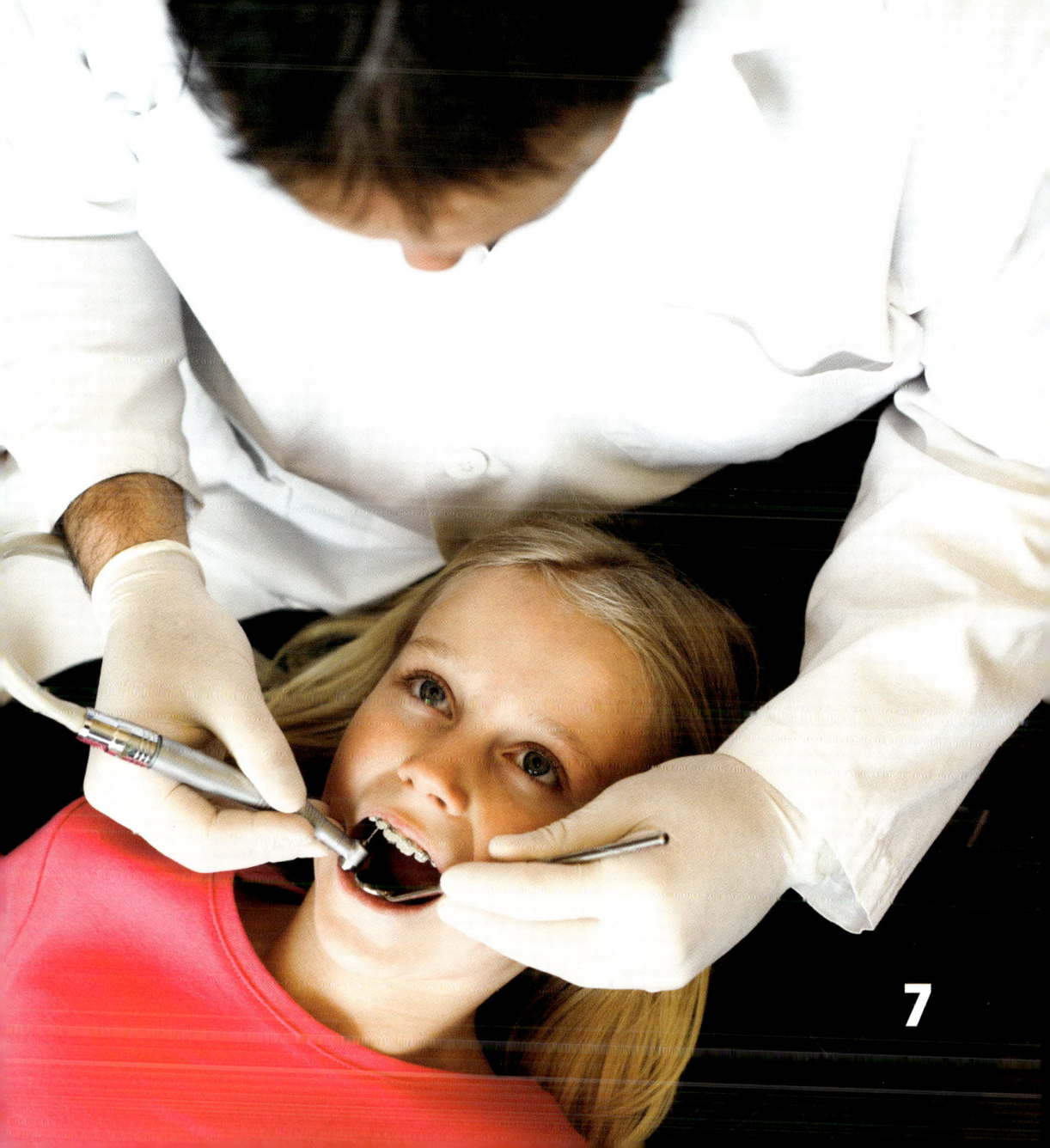

7

I need to see inside your mouth.

I check your teeth for **decay**.

You have to open wide!

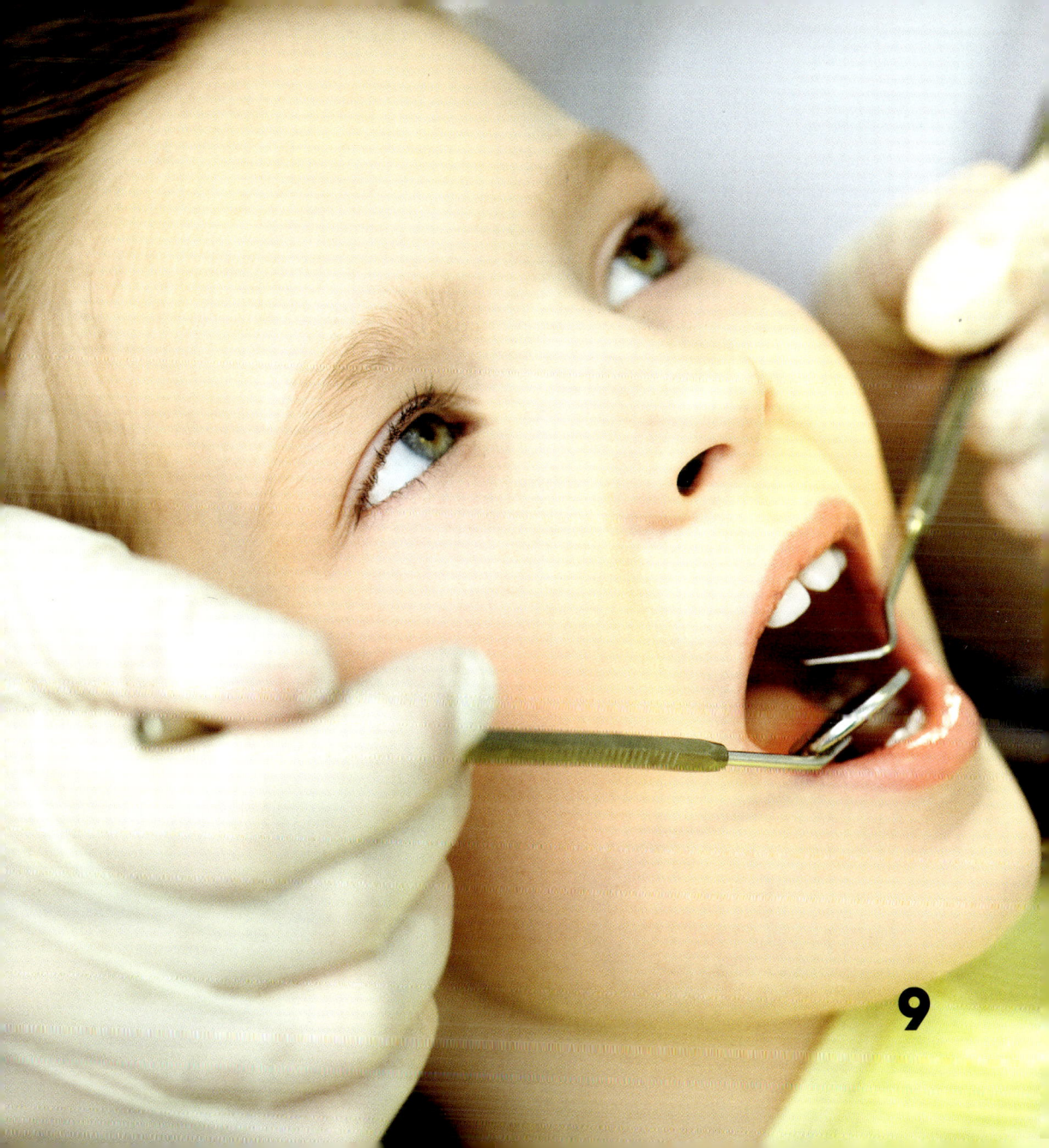

9

I take **X-rays** of your mouth.

This helps me find **cavities**.

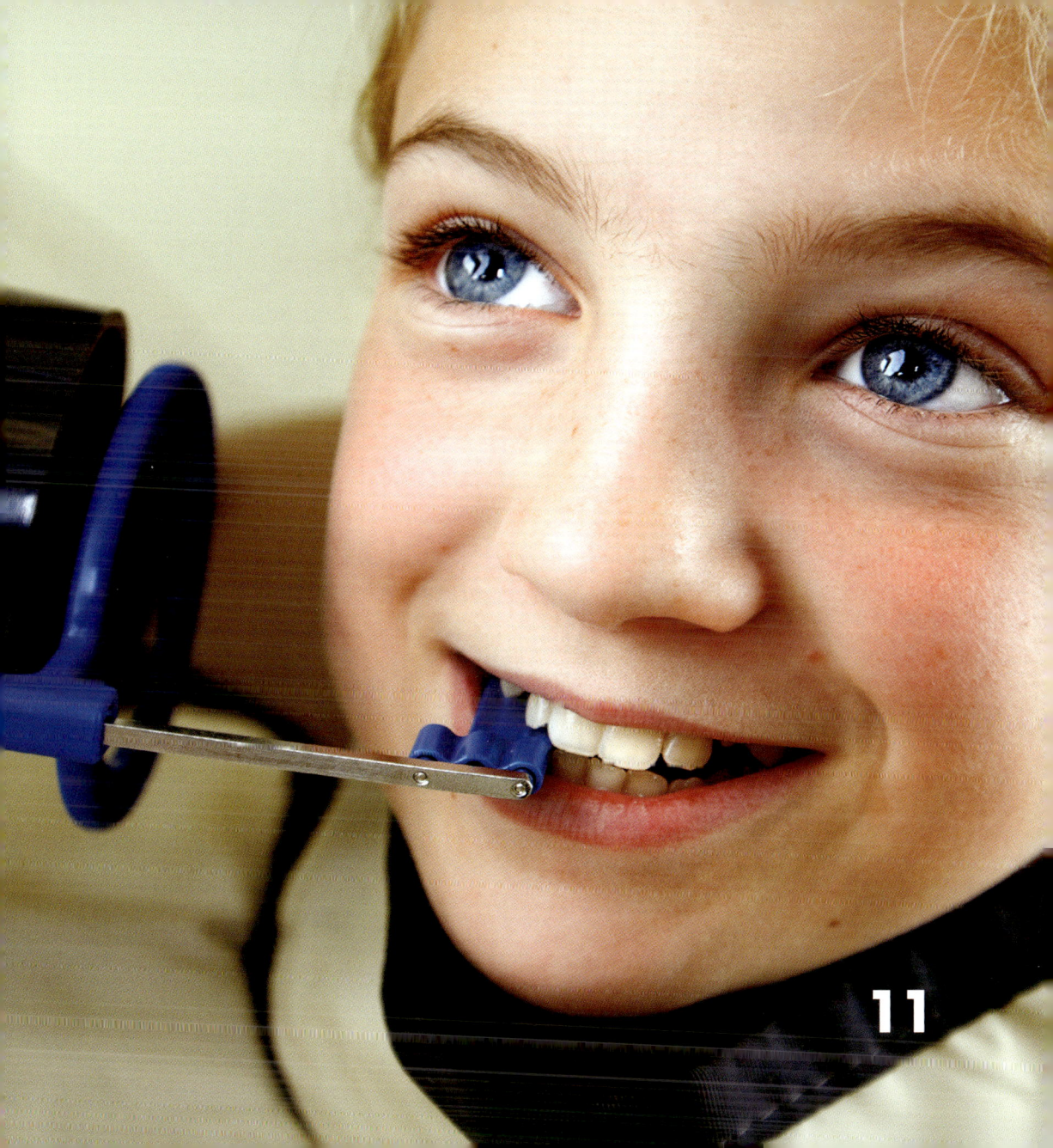

I use a mirror and special tools to check your teeth.

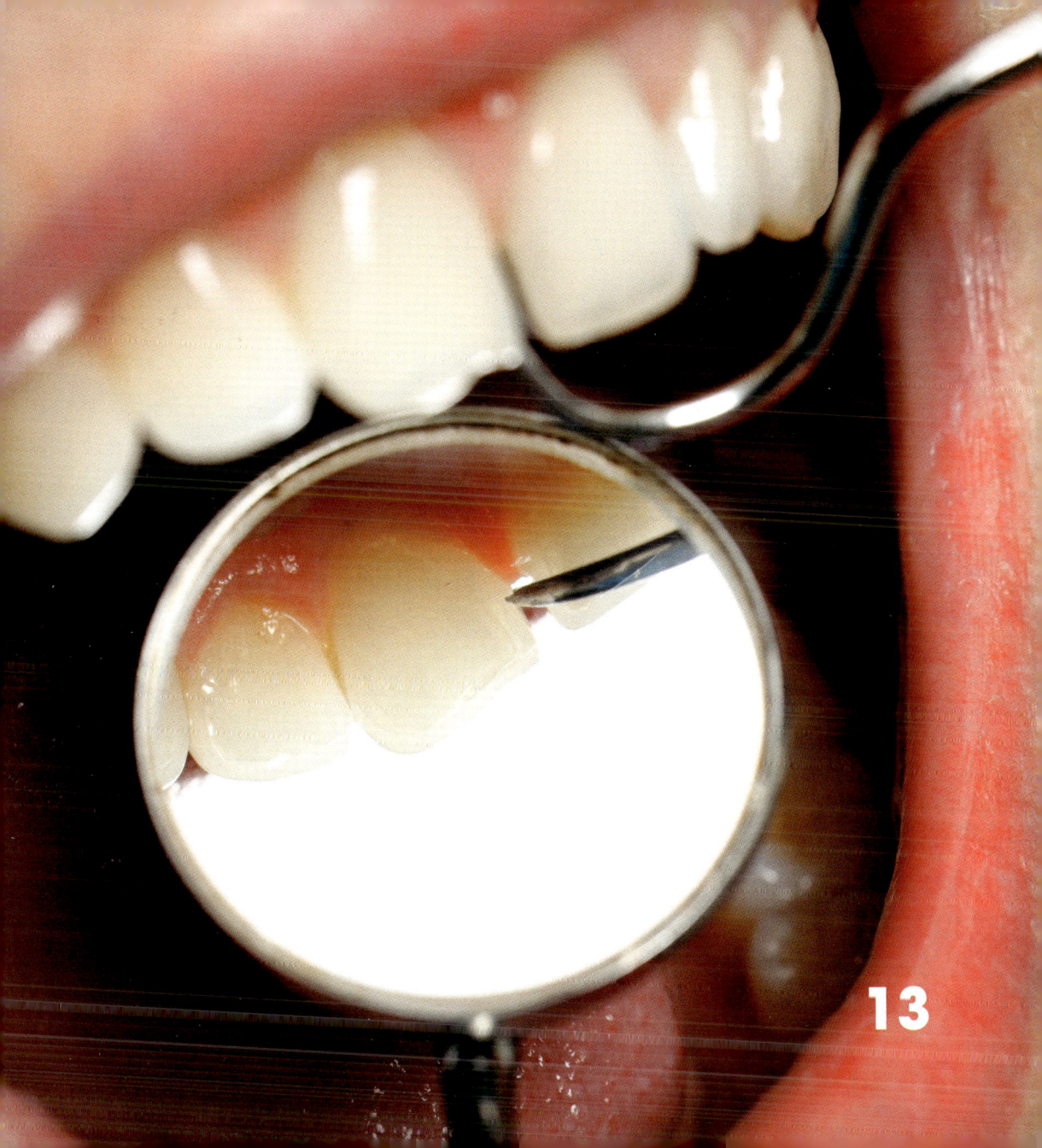

I fix any cavities I find.

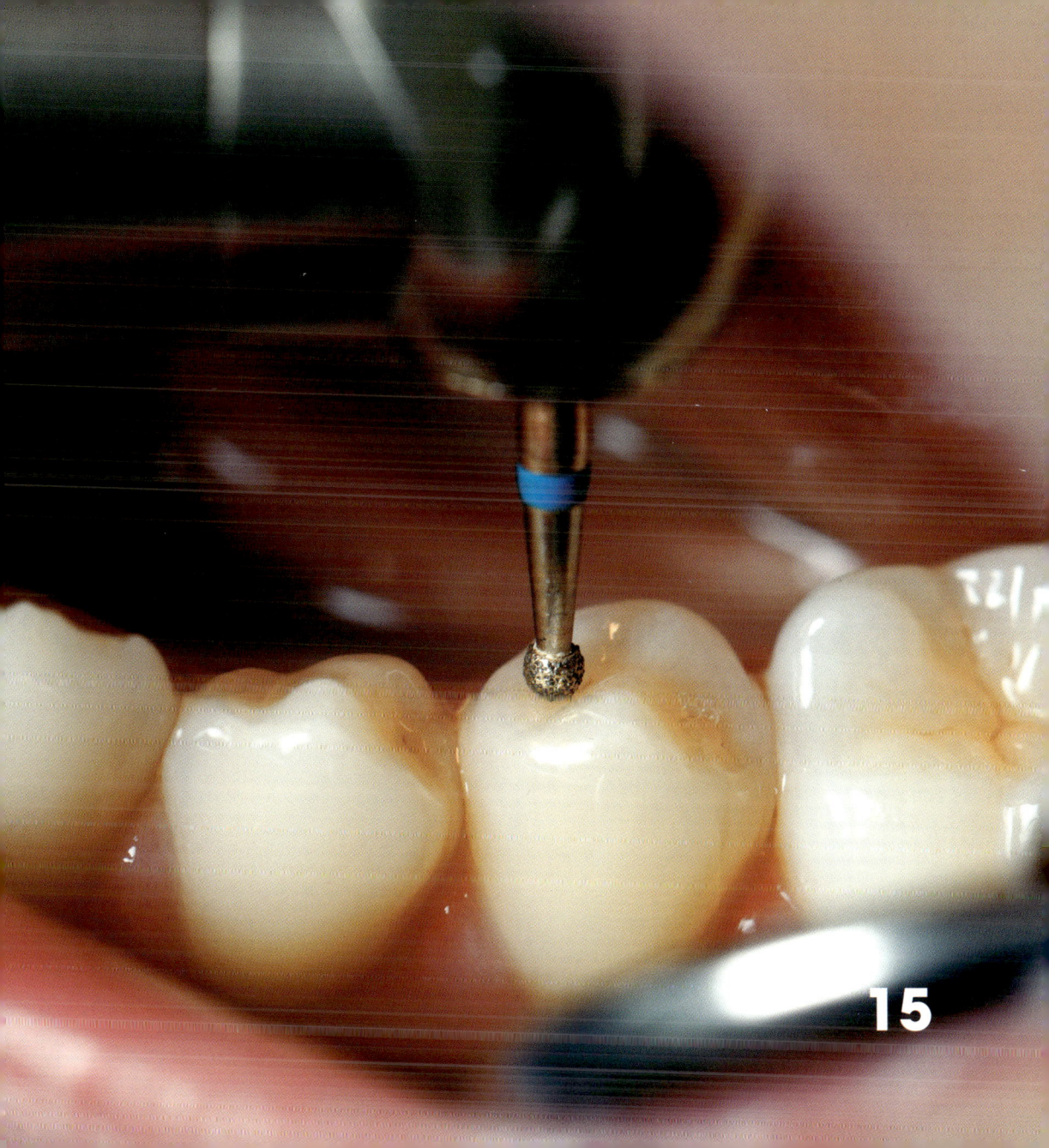

I will show you how to brush your teeth.

Then, I will show you how to **floss**.

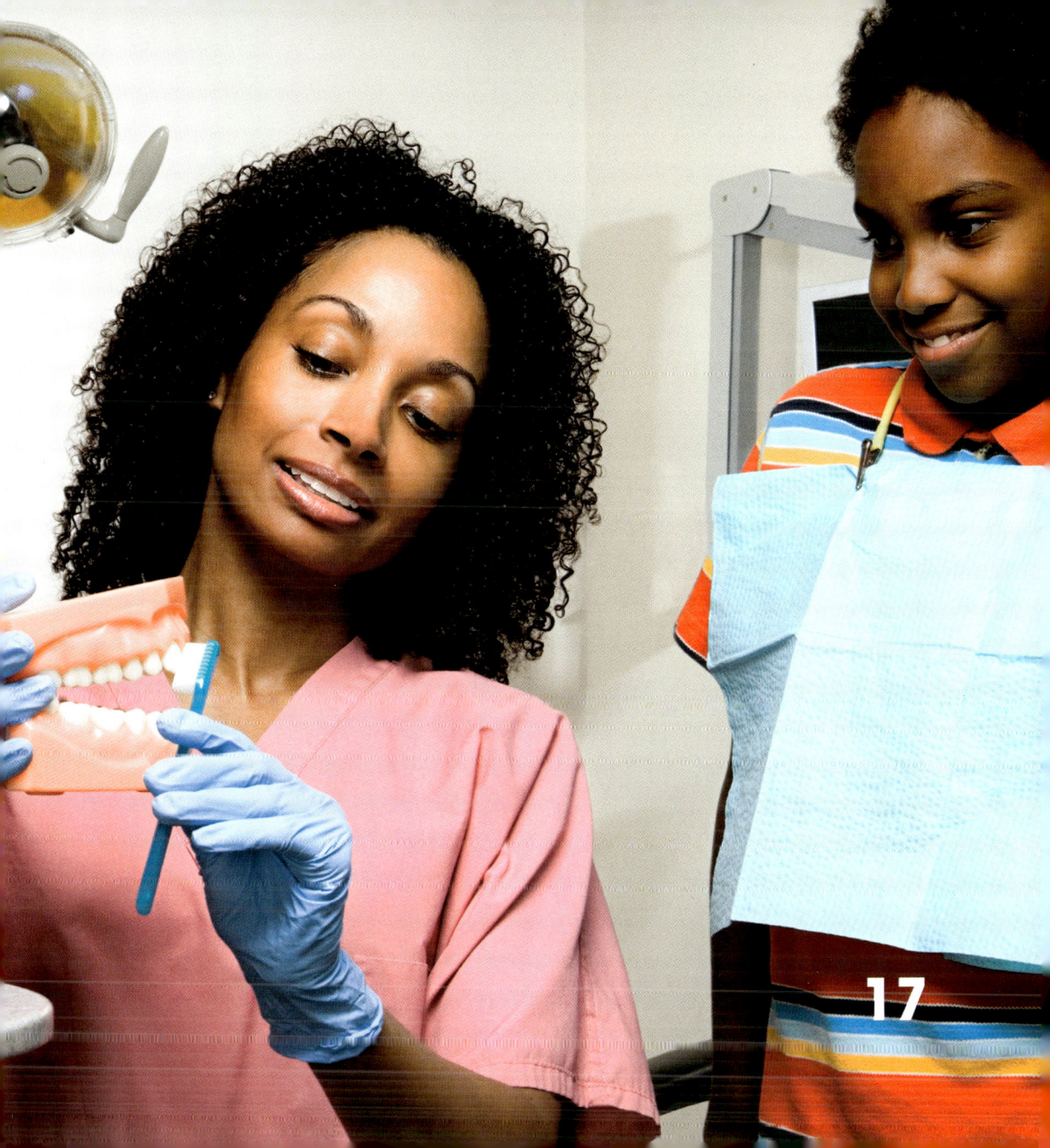
17

Your teeth look good!

Here is a new toothbrush.

It will keep your teeth clean and healthy.

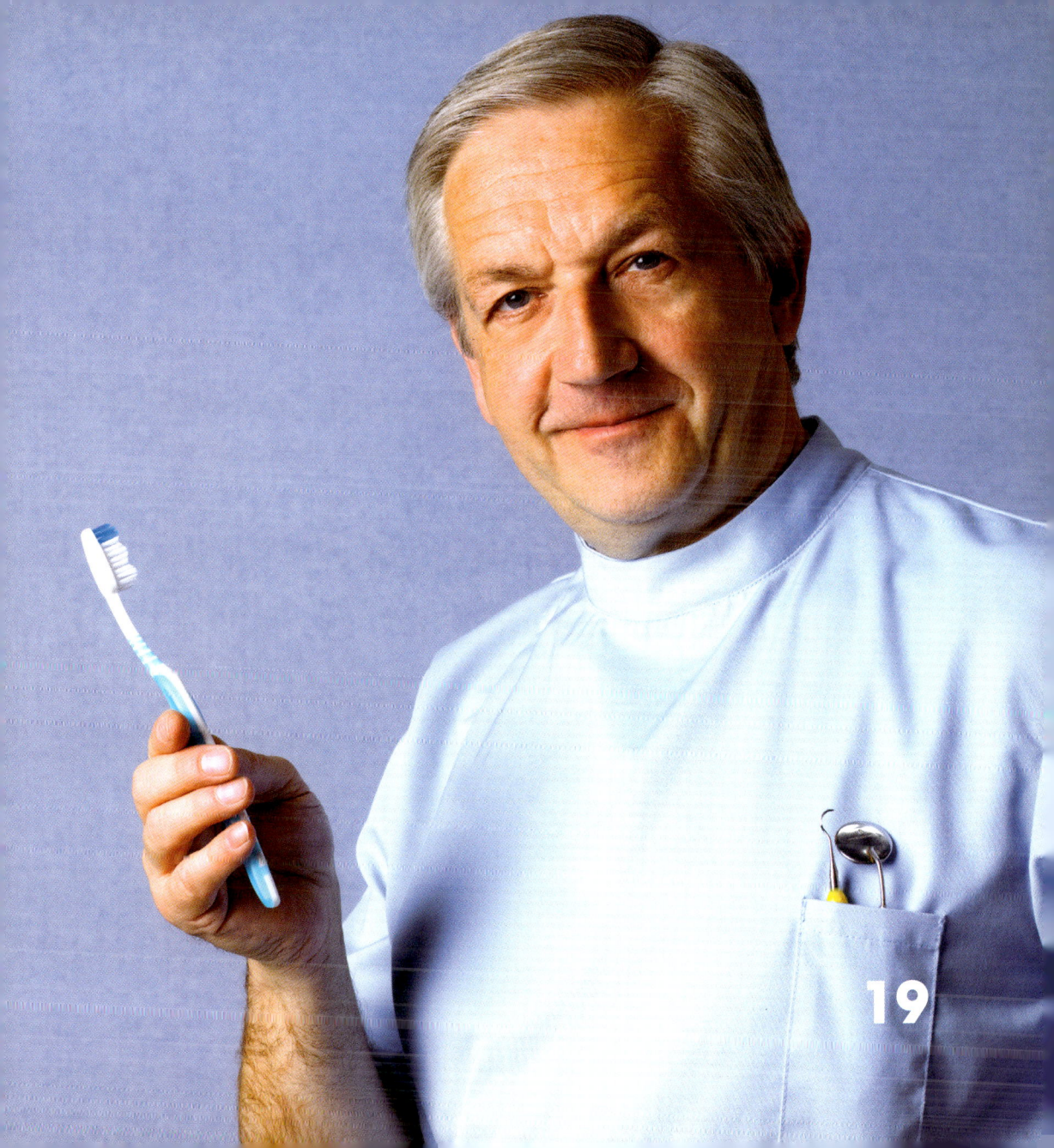

Don't forget to brush and eat right.

See you in six months!

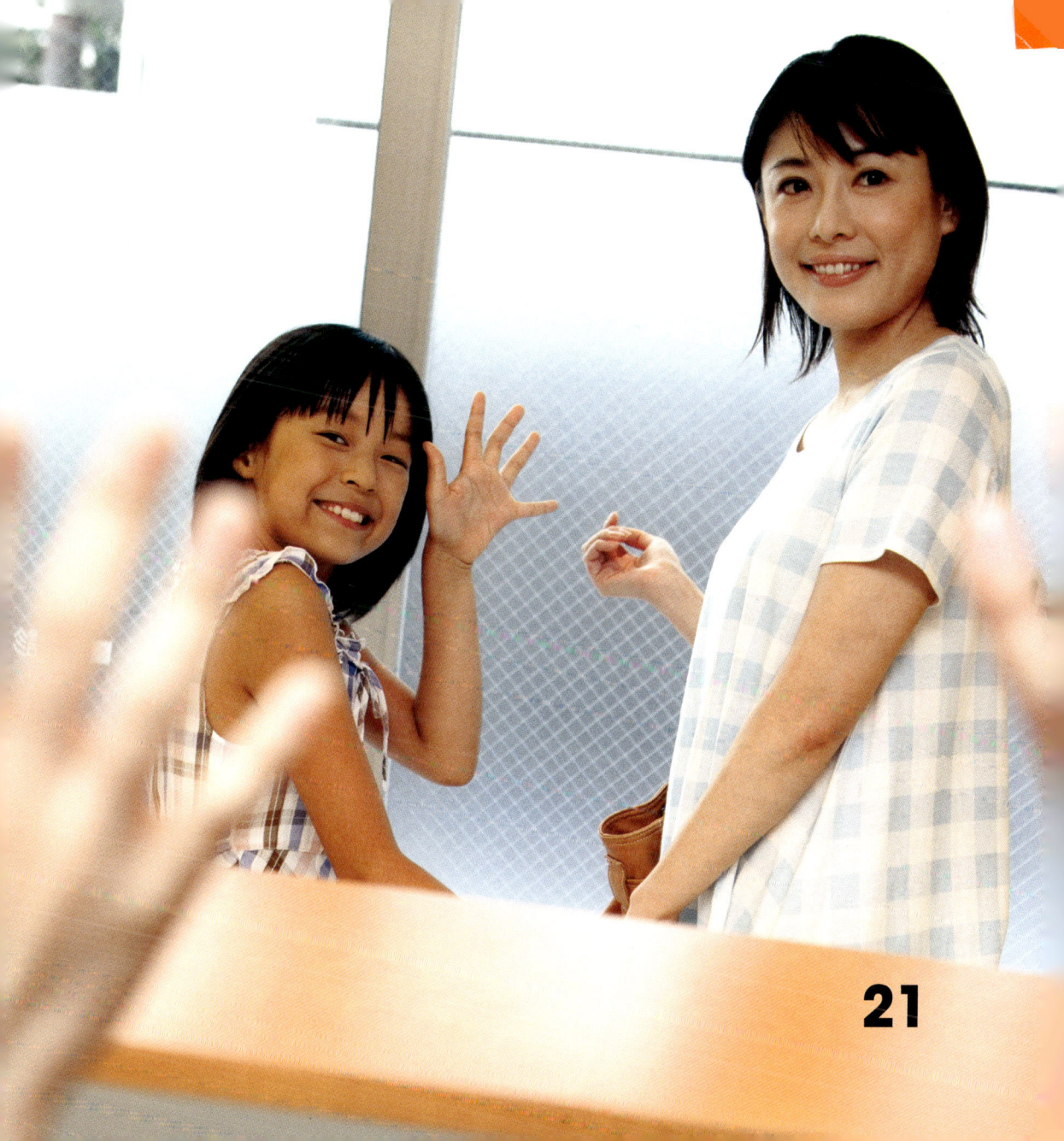
21

New Words

cavities (KAV-e-teez) Holes on the inside or outside of your teeth.

decay (dee-K) The wearing away of the surface or the inside of your teeth.

floss (FLOSS) To clean between your teeth with dental floss.

healthy (HEL-thee) To be without sickness or damage.

X-rays (X-rayz) Pictures of teeth or bones inside our body.

Index

cavities, 10, 14

decay, 8

floss, 16

healthy, 4, 18

X-rays, 10

About the Author

Erika de Nijs played college hockey before becoming a teacher and a writer. Her parents are from the Netherlands but she was raised in Upstate New York.

About BOOKWORMS

Bookworms help independent readers gain reading confidence through high-frequency words, simple sentences, and strong picture/text support. Each book explores a concept that helps children relate what they read to the world in which they live.